A CLINI
THE

A CLINICAL PHARMACOLOGY AND THERAPEUTICS CATECHISM

Howard J. Rogers
MA, MB, BChir, PhD, FRCP

Professor of Clinical Pharmacology
United Medical and Dental Schools of
Guy's and St Thomas's Hospitals,
London

Roy G. Spector
MD, PhD, FRCP, FRCPath

Professor of Applied Pharmacology
United Medical and Dental Schools of
Guy's and St Thomas's Hospitals,
London

HODDER AND STOUGHTON

LONDON SYDNEY AUCKLAND TORONTO

British Library Cataloguing in Publication Data

Rogers, H. J.
A clinical pharmacology and therapeutics catechism.
1. Chemotherapy – Examinations, questions, etc.
I. Title II. Spector, R. G.
615.5'8'076 RM262

ISBN 0 340 40147 8

First published 1986

Typeset by Rowland Phototypesetting Ltd,
Bury St Edmunds, Suffolk

Printed in Great Britain for Hodder and Stoughton Educational,
a division of Hodder and Stoughton Ltd, Mill Road, Dunton Green,
Sevenoaks, Kent TN13 2YD, by Richard Clay Ltd, Bungay, Suffolk

CONTENTS

INTRODUCTION

In many of the medical qualifying examinations, separate sections are now devoted to clinical pharmacology and therapeutics. This is not surprising considering that the majority of consultations between doctors and patients result in the prescription of drugs or the modification of drug treatment.

Although the subject of drug science is now vast, the scope of the *viva voce* examination in clinical pharmacology and therapeutics is more restricted. In over a decade of involvement with the London final MB exams (and other similar qualifying examinations), we have come to the conclusion that the most important function of the *viva* is to provide a finer discrimination in performance than that given by the written papers alone. We feel that the most revealing questions are not difficult or complex, but test knowledge of straightforward and widely accepted treatments of common medical conditions. The majority of these diseases are frequently seen in any medical clinic or represent important examples of acute illness in which drugs make a useful contribution to treatment. However questions also come up on rarities which are good examination fodder, and which the examiners cannot resist because they demonstrate pharmacological principles so well. Thus myasthenia gravis and the cheese reaction keep appearing in exams.

In this little book we have collected together the most frequently asked questions that we have come across in this subject in the final MB orals. For the sake of brevity and convenience we have not used the exact verbal style of the questions – in which one short question and answer leads to several more on the same topic – but condensed such a sequence into a rather more substantial single question and answer.

PHARMACOKINETICS, PHARMACODYNAMICS AND GENERAL PHARMACOLOGY

Q1 What is pharmacokinetics?

A The study of all the factors which control the concentration of drugs in the body. These include drug absorption, distribution metabolism and excretion.

Q2 What is the distinction between pharmacokinetics and pharmacodynamics?

A Pharmacokinetics is what the body does to drugs: pharmacodynamics is what drugs do to the body.

Q3 What is meant by the term 'half life' of a drug?

A This is the elimination half life. It is the time taken for the concentration in the blood to fall by half. It is measured after drug absorption and redistribution have been completed.

Q4 What is the steady state level?

A When a drug is repeatedly administered a situation is reached when the amount of drug absorbed is equal to that lost by elimination. It is attained after approximately 5 half lives of the drug.

Q5 What is the apparent volume of distribution?

A Drugs are distributed in body fluids and adsorbed on body structures to different extents. Thus the concentration in the plasma may not represent the concentration of the drug in other parts of the body. The apparent volume of distribution is an artificial arithmetical concept relating to the amount of drug administered and its apparent dilution in the body fluids as evidenced by its concentration in the blood. It is calculated by dividing the amount of drug in the body by the concentration reached in the plasma.

Q6 What is clearance?

A Clearance is a measure of drug elimination and is expressed as the volume of plasma from which all drug is removed in unit time.

It can be calculated as:

$$\text{clearance} = \frac{0.7 \times \text{volume of distribution}}{\text{half life}}$$

Q7 What is bioavailability?

A This is a measure of the proportion of an administered dose of a drug which is taken up by the body. Failure to take up 100% of a dose may be due to incomplete absorption or to first pass metabolism by the liver or gut.

Q8 What is the meaning of the term 'first order elimination kinetics'?

A This is when a constant proportion of the drug remaining in the body is eliminated in unit time. This happens when the rate of elimination at any moment is proportional to the amount of drug in the body at that time.

First order elimination produces an exponential decay in drug concentration in the blood when plotted against time. The rate of decay can be expressed as a half life.

Q9 What is the meaning of the term 'zero order elimination kinetics'?

A This is when the rate of elimination is constant (and independent of how much drug remains in the body). There is no single half life value to describe this but the elimination rate can be expressed as a constant weight of drug eliminated/kg bodyweight/hour.

Zero order elimination happens when a drug is given in an amount which exceeds the maximum capacity of the elimination mechanism in the body.

Q10 Describe the difference between potency and efficacy.

A Potency is a weight-for-weight comparison of how much of different drugs must be given to obtain the same effect.

Efficacy is a comparison of the therapeutic effect of different drugs when given in optimal doses.

Q11 Give examples of some indications for estimating plasma levels of drugs.

A (a) Lithium: this always should be done as there is a clear therapeutic range which is narrow and which is attained with different doses in different individuals.

(b) In renal failure: drugs which have dose-dependent toxicity and are mainly eliminated by the kidneys may accumulate dangerously in renal failure. Examples include aminoglycoside antibiotics and digoxin.

(c) Phenytoin: it is sometimes helpful to perform blood levels because phenytoin is eliminated by zero order kinetics and thus the relationship between steady state blood levels and daily dose is not linear – small increments of dose may produce large increases in blood level.

(d) In any situation when failure of compliance is suspected.

Q12 Which types of drug interaction are of most clinical importance?

A (a) When drugs are involved which produce important clinical consequences when their effects are slightly increased or decreased (i.e., drugs with a low therapeutic ratio). Examples include contraceptive pill failure after inducing agents have been administered; haemorrhage from warfarin after highly protein bound drugs given as well; hypoglycaemia from tolbutamide if its hepatic metabolism is inhibited with a large dose of alcohol; digoxin toxicity following hypokalaemia produced by diuretics.

(b) Drugs eliminated by zero order kinetics are sensitive to small changes in their rate of elimination. For example, phenytoin toxicity can develop if isoniazid is added to the regime because of inhibition of metabolism of phenytoin.

(c) Central nervous system depressants potentiate each other, e.g., alcohol and benzodiazepines.

(d) Specific interactions:

(i) alcohol can produce a disulfiram type action in patients taking sulphonylureas or metronidazole.

(ii) allopurinol blocks the metabolism of mercaptopurine and so increases its toxicity.

(iii) amphetamine and similar sympathomimetic amines can cause a hypertensive reaction in patients taking monoamine oxidase inhibitors.

Q13 What are some of the problems caused by drugs in the newborn?

A (a) Immaturity of drug metabolising enzyme systems, e.g., chloramphenicol is not conjugated with glucuronic acid and large amounts of the non-conjugated drug can cause the grey syndrome.

(b) If the child is jaundiced then highly protein bound drugs (e.g., sulphonamides) can displace bilirubin from albumin and cause kernicterus.

(c) Some drugs are excreted in the milk, e.g., opioids, senna, benzodiazepines.

(d) The newborn child can suffer withdrawal states if the mother abused drugs during pregnancy.

Q14 What are some of the common difficulties in drug administration to the elderly?

A (a) Pharmacokinetic: metabolism may be reduced, e.g., lignocaine, propranolol, amylobarbitone. Excretion may be reduced, e.g., digoxin, aminoglycosides, lithium.

(b) Pharmacodynamic: for example, tricyclic antidepressants have more severe and more dangerous anticholinergic actions; digoxin and benztropine are more likely to produce acute psychotic reactions; diuretics and neuroleptics have a greater tendency to cause severe postural hypotension; hypnotics may produce nocturnal confusion.

(c) Compliance failure may be commoner in the elderly because of communication difficulties.

Q15 What are the problems of being a slow or fast acetylator?

A Fast acetylators require higher, and sometimes more frequent, doses of isoniazid, procainamide, hydralazine. Slow acetylators develop toxicity more frequently with isoniazid (peripheral neuropathy), procainamide and hydralazine (anti-nuclear antibodies and systemic lupus), phenelzine (liver damage) and sulphasalazine (red cell damage). However, isoniazid hepatitis is more common among fast acetylators.

Sulphapyridine → N+V, Headache, Rash

THE NERVOUS SYSTEM, PAIN AND RHEUMATISM

Q1 What is a hypnotic drug?

A A substance which can induce sleep. The sleep produced resembles physiological sleep in that the patient can be roused by external stimuli, but may be abnormal in that dreaming may be suppressed, the electroencephalogram is altered and the patient may not recover normal cerebral function for several hours after wakening.

Q2 What are the disadvantages of using hypnotics?

A
(a) Dependence – discontinuation producing anxiety, insomnia and distressing, vivid dreams.
(b) Respiratory depression – particularly in emphysematous and asthmatic subjects and in those who take alcohol at night.
(c) Falls in the elderly.
(d) Confusion and delirium in the elderly.
(e) Hangover.
(f) Special problems (e.g., gastritis and rashes with chloral; enzyme induction with dichloralphenazone; anticholinergic activity with promethazine).

Q3 Describe benzodiazepine dependence. In other words, what happens on drug withdrawal?

A
(a) Anxiety, panic attacks, insomnia, increased dreaming.
(b) Decreased appetite, dyspepsia.
(c) Fits.
(d) Pains: headaches, muscle ache, muscle spasms.
(e) Hyperperception: increased sensitivity to touch and painful stimuli, hyperacusis, photophobia, hyperosmia.

(f) Abnormal perception: the patient feels as if he is covered in cotton wool or walking on a thick carpet; vertigo.
(g) Depression.

Q4 How may the benzodiazepines be classified?

A (a) Longer acting with long-lived active metabolites, e.g., diazepam ($t_{1/2}$ 20–50h) has a metabolite demethyldiazepam ($t_{1/2}$ 100h).
(b) Shorter acting with no long-lived active metabolites, e.g., temazepam ($t_{1/2}$ 5–20h).

Q5 What are the main long-term medical consequences of repeated administration of large amounts of ethanol?

A (a) Dependence: tremor, fits and DTs on withdrawal.
(b) Dementia due to direct cerebral damage. Depression and suicide.
(c) Korsakov's psychosis and Wernicke's encephalopathy due to thiamine deficiency: other vitamin deficiencies.
(d) Alimentary diseases: gastritis, peptic ulcer, pancreatitis, cirrhosis of the liver, alcoholic hepatitis.
(e) Fetal alcohol syndrome.
(f) Cardiomyopathy.

Q6 What drugs interact with alcohol?

A (a) Sedatives – potentiation of sedation and respiratory depression.
(b) NSAIDs – potentiation of gastric irritation.
(c) Hypoglycaemic agents – potentiation of hypoglycaemia.
(d) Anticoagulants – gastric haemorrhage.
(e) Aldehyde dehydrogenase inhibitors, e.g., metronidazole – antabuse-like reaction.

Q7 How may drugs be used in the treatment of Parkinson's disease?

A The condition arises from a deficiency in dopamine transmission in the extrapyramidal system, thus the balance of cholinergic (excitatory) and dopaminergic (inhibitory) systems is disturbed. The treatment strategies include:

(a) Reduce cholinergic actions with acetylcholine receptor blockers such as benzhexol.

(b) Increase dopamine-like effects:

(i) by giving the dopamine precursor, levodopa. Dopamine itself does not penetrate the blood brain barrier but levodopa enters the brain and is then decarboxylated to form dopamine.

(ii) other dopamine receptor agonists include bromocriptine.

(iii) increase dopamine release from nerves by administering amantadine.

(iv) reduce dopamine metabolism with a monoamine oxidase B inhibitor (selegiline).

Q8 What are the hazards of levodopa treatment?

A (a) Nausea and vomiting.

(b) Postural hypotension.

(c) Cardiac arrhythmias.

(d) Motor disturbances: dystonias, motor restlessness, chorea, painful cramps, on-off phenomena.

(e) Psychiatric effects: vivid dreams, depression, hallucinations, psychotic episodes. One third of patients with Parkinson's disease treated this way develop dementia.

Q9 How may these toxic effects be reduced?

A A decarboxylase inhibitor given with levodopa reduces the incidence and severity of nausea and of cardiac arrhythmias.

Selegiline with levodopa and a decarboxylase inhibitor may reduce on-off phenomena and some dyskinesias.

Q10 Outline the use of drugs in migraine.

A (a) The acute attack usually responds to an analgesic such as aspirin or paracetamol. Metoclopramide may be required 15 minutes before these drugs if nausea is present.

Ergotamine tartrate may terminate attacks which have not responded to analgesics.

(b) Prophylactic therapy may be tried for several months in patients who experience two or more attacks each month. The most widely used prophylactic drugs are pizotifen (a 5-HT and histamine (H_1) receptor blocker), and propranolol (a β adrenoceptor blocker).

Q11 What are the dangers of ergotamine?

A
(a) An excessive dose can cause giddiness, nausea and headache, which may cause the patient to think the migraine requires more drug.
(b) Large doses produce vasospasm leading to gangrene of the fingers and toes and myocardial ischaemia.
(c) Mental and neurological changes.
(d) Abortion.

Q12 In a patient with myasthenia gravis, how may one distinguish between a myasthenic and cholinergic crisis?

A Patients with myasthenia gravis may become weaker because of over-treatment – particularly with a powerful long-acting anticholinesterase such as distigmine – (cholinergic crisis) or because the disease itself has worsened (myasthenic crisis) and requires a higher dose of anticholinesterase. The two conditions can be distinguished with a very short-acting anticholinesterase, edrophonium. This will cause a transient improvement in muscle power during a myasthenic crisis, but will cause no effect or a deterioration in a cholinergic crisis.

Q13 Outline the main principles of drug therapy in the management of terminal pain.

A
(a) It may not be necessary to commence with opioids, or to use these exclusively. Aspirin and similar drugs (e.g., indomethacin, naproxen) may be tried initially or in combination with opioids.
(b) Whenever possible give opioids by mouth or by suppository. Try codeine or dihydrocodeine before co-proxamol, then phenazocine and finally morphine or diamorphine (or a similar sequence of other opioids).

(c) A dose is given which is sufficient to relieve pain, and is repeated at an interval such that the pain does not recur. Pain itself lowers the pain threshold. The drugs are not prescribed 'p.r.n.'.

(d) If injections of powerful opioids are used, diamorphine is preferred to morphine because it can be dissolved in a smaller volume of solution.

(e) Other drugs can be given with opioids, including cyclizine or metoclopramide (for nausea); chlorpromazine (for confusion, nausea or to enhance the tranquilliser action of the opioid); amitriptyline (for depression); docusate (for opioid-induced constipation); diazepam (for anxiety).

Q14 What types of drugs are used in treating rheumatoid arthritis?

A (a) Non-steroidal anti-inflammatory drugs (e.g., aspirin, indomethacin, naproxen).

(b) Local or systemic steroids (e.g., prednisolone).

(c) Drugs which affect the disease process (gold, penicillamine, chloroquine and other immunosuppressive and immunopotentiating drugs).

Q15 What are the common toxic effects of indomethacin?

A (a) The toxic effects shared by the non-steroidal anti-inflammatory analgesics include:

(i) dyspepsia, gastritis, gastric and duodenal haemorrhage from pre-existing peptic ulcer; haemorrhage from the stomach if anticoagulants, alcohol and glucocorticoids are given concurrently.

(ii) aggravation of asthma in some atopic individuals. Also urticaria and other rashes can result.

(iii) overdose produces respiratory alkalosis followed by metabolic acidosis with aspirin. Indomethacin can also produce metabolic and electrolyte disturbances.

(iv) dose-dependent toxicity induces giddiness, nausea and tinnitus.

(v) fluid retention.

(vi) delay onset of labour and possible other adverse effects in pregnancy.
(vii) probably all members of the group can cause renal and hepatic damage.

(b) Effects peculiar to indomethacin are giddiness, headaches and confusion.

Q16 What precautions are required when sodium aurothiomalate is given?

A (a) Treatment is stopped if proteinuria develops.
(b) RBC, WBC and platelet counts are performed before each injection, to detect bone marrow depression. The treatment is stopped if any value is depressed.
(c) If a rash develops, treatment is temporarily withdrawn.

Q17 What drugs can be used to treat gout?

A (a) Acute attacks can be treated with colchicine given 4-hourly till relief or diarrhoea occurs. The NSAIDs are usually less toxic; indomethacin or naproxen may terminate an attack. Severe refractory episodes usually respond to steroids.
(b) If recurrent attacks occur, then hypouricaemic drugs are given. These include the uricosurics (probenecid and sulphinpyrazone) and the xanthine oxidase inhibitors (e.g., allopurinol). Both of these types of prophylactic therapy can cause a temporary exacerbation of the acute attacks. Because of this a non-steroidal anti-inflammatory drug should be given concurrently during the first few months of treatment.

Q18 Which drugs are useful in the management of the various clinical types of epilepsy?

A The anti-epileptic drugs can be grouped according to their effectiveness in the different forms of epilepsy:
(a) Petit mal absences with a 3 Hz spike and wave EEG: ethosuximide, clonazepam, sodium valproate.
(b) Myoclonic seizures and akinetic attacks: clonazepam, sodium valproate.
(c) Salaam attacks with hypsarrhythmia: nitrazepam, glucocorticoids or corticotrophin.

(d) Tonic clonic fits, focal fits and temporal lobe epilepsy: carbamazepine, phenytoin, sodium valproate, primidone, phenobarbitone.

Q19 Outline the factors you would consider before deciding to start anti-convulsant therapy.

A (a) How many attacks have occurred?

(b) Are the attacks true fits (i.e., as opposed to hysteria, breath holding attacks, sleep paralysis)?

(c) If this is true epilepsy, is there a cause which requires treatment (e.g., tumour, granuloma, hypocalcaemia)?

(d) If no cause is detected are there precipitating factors which can be avoided (e.g., disco lights, fluorescent tubes, hunger, alcohol)?

(e) What is the clinical and EEG type of epilepsy – so that an appropriate drug might be prescribed if the decision is made to start anti-convulsant therapy?

Q20 Which types of drug are used in myasthenia gravis?

A (a) Anticholinesterases:

(i) neostigmine – action lasts up to 4 hours. Muscarinic actions are pronounced (e.g., colic, salivation, bronchial secretion) but can be reduced with atropine.

(ii) pyridostigmine – more prolonged action.

(b) Corticosteroids, when thymectomy cannot be carried out.

(c) When corticosteroids are used, azathioprine usually produces additional benefit.

Q21 What is the cheese reaction and how can it be treated?

A Patients who are taking monoamine oxidase inhibitors (MAOI) for depression develop a severe hypertensive reaction if they eat cheese. This is called the cheese reaction and is due to the tyramine content of cheese. Tyramine is normally destroyed by the amineoxidases in the intestinal epithelium and liver. When these oxidases are blocked by MAOI, dietary tyramine enters the circulation and acts as an indirectly acting sympathomimetic drug – in other words it displaces stores of noradrenaline and adrenaline from sympathetic nerve endings and the adrenal medulla. Such stores are augmented in patients taking MAOI and thus large amounts of catecholamines are liberated causing hypertension, tachycardia and hyperthermia. The condition is treated with an α-receptor blocker (e.g., ~~chlorpromazine~~) and a β-blocker (e.g., propranolol).

phentolamine

CARDIOVASCULAR DISEASE

Q1 Outline the treatment of acute left ventricular failure.

A
(a) The patient is nursed in the sitting position and 100% oxygen is administered if there is no chronic obstructive respiratory disease.
(b) Whenever possible the precipitating cause is treated. Thus severe hypertension may be treated with systemic labetalol or hydralazine. Intravenous sodium nitroprusside may be used if the facilities of an intensive care unit are available. However the blood pressure should not be lowered precipitously.
(c) Intravenous frusemide or bumetanide is given to relieve the severe dyspnoea due to pulmonary oedema.
(d) Morphine reduces the sensation of dyspnoea, reduces excessive respiratory effort and reduces the work of the heart (by venodilatation and reducing afterload).
(e) Many physicians also administer aminophylline as a bronchodilator.

Q2 How is moderately severe essential hypertension managed?

A
(a) General measures: stop smoking, reduce obesity, look for and control diabetes mellitus, treat hyperlipidaemia. Physical exercise and relaxation therapy may be beneficial. Dietary salt restriction is not universally recommended.
(b) Treatment may be started with a β-blocker or diuretic or a combination of the two. If the response to the combination is not adequate, a vasodilator (e.g., hydralazine) or calcium antagonist (e.g., nifedipine) or α_1 blocker (e.g., prazosin) may be added.

Nifedipine or prazosin can be used on their own. An angiotensin converting enzyme inhibitor (e.g., captopril) is useful in moderate to severe hypertension and is usually given with a loop diuretic (e.g., frusemide).

Q3 What are the main toxic effects of the β-blockers?

A
(a) Severe bronchospasm in patients with asthma, bronchitis or chronic rhinitis.
(b) Precipitation of heart failure.
(c) Loss of ability to exercise, reduced physical energy.
(d) Increased danger of severe hypoglycaemia in diabetics treated with hypoglycaemic agents.
(e) Cold extremities, Raynaud's phenomena.
(f) Nightmares and vivid dreams.

Q4 What are the main uses of β-blockers?

A
(a) Cardiovascular disease – especially hypertension, angina pectoris and protection against myocardial reinfarction.
(b) Nervous system – migraine prophylaxis and reduction in peripheral manifestation of anxiety (e.g., palpitations and tremor).
(c) Hyperthyroidism (reduction in sympathetic manifestation, e.g., atrial tachycardia and atrial fibrillation).
(d) Eye drops (timolol) in glaucoma.

Q5 Outline the management of a lady aged 45 who presents in your clinic complaining of a severe headache for the past week. You find she has a sitting blood pressure of 250/150 mm Hg and that she has papilloedema.

A
(a) The patient should be immediately admitted to hospital for investigation and to initiate treatment.
(b) The blood pressure is lowered, but care is taken that the fall is not precipitous. Malignant (accelerated) hypertension is not in itself an indication for parenteral drug therapy. Labetalol (or metoprolol) with or without hydralazine or nifedipine by mouth may be successful. If the response is not satisfactory

over 2 or 3 days then other drug combinations may be tried – these include diuretics with other vasodilators or angiotensin converting enzyme blockers.

(c) If a more rapid fall in blood pressure is required then intravenous labetalol or hydralazine may be used. If the facilities of an intensive care unit are available then intravenous sodium nitroprusside can be infused.

Q6 How do the main types of anti-anginal drugs act?

A (a) The nitrates and nitrites cause dilatation of the capacitance vessels by acting directly on peripheral venules. This causes reduced venous return, hence reduced diastolic filling of the ventricles and diminished work performed by the myocardium. These drugs may also dilate the coronary vessels and reduce peripheral (arteriolar) resistance.

(b) The β adrenoceptor blockers prevent the increased oxygen requirement by the myocardium during exercise and emotional excitement by preventing the sympathetic nervous system and adrenal medullary hormones stimulating the cardiac (β_1) receptors.

(c) The calcium antagonists reduce peripheral resistance by dilating arterioles (especially nifedipine), reducing supraventricular pacemaker activity (especially verapamil) and directly dilating coronary arteries. Verapamil may also have a quinidine-like effect on the myocardium and decrease its work and oxygen consumption.

RENAL SYSTEM AND METABOLIC DISEASE

Q1 Which drugs cause particular problems when given to patients with chronic renal failure?

A (a) Substances eliminated by the kidneys which have a low therapeutic index, e.g., aminoglycosides, nitrofurantoin, digoxin, ethambutol.

(b) Agents causing nausea, e.g., theophylline.

(c) Antianabolic agents which can aggravate uraemia, e.g., tetracyclines, glucocorticoids.

(d) Agents metabolised by the kidneys, e.g., failure to activate vitamin D.

Q2 How may the excretion of drugs be promoted?

A (a) Forced diuresis (by giving fluids or diuretics) reduces renal reabsorption by speeding transit through the renal tubules.

(b) Acidifying the urine (increases ionisation of bases such as pethidine and amphetamine); alkalinising the urine (increases the ionisation of acids such as aspirin and barbiturates). Ionised drugs are not reabsorbed via the renal tubules.

(c) Dialysis (if the drug is diffusible and not extensively tissue bound).

Q3 What are the hazards of the thiazide diuretics?

A (a) Hypokalaemia, especially in the elderly or in patients with chronic heart failure, but not usually in patients treated for hypertension.

(b) Reduced glucose tolerance.

(c) Hyperuricaemia.

(d) Impotence.

(e) Raised plasma cholesterol.

(f) Hypochloraemic alkalosis.
(g) Uncommonly, rashes and thrombocytopenia.

Q4 Outline the main strategies in the management of hyperglycaemic coma in a diabetic.

A
(a) Initial and general measures: admit to hospital and insert venous cannula. General care of the unconscious patient includes insertion of nasogastric tube and bladder catheter. Send sample of blood to laboratory (glucose, ketones, pH, pCO_2 blood culture, electrolytes). Repeat hourly.
(b) Assess precipitating cause and treat if appropriate (e.g., infection, trauma, infarction, stroke).
(c) Correct dehydration, using intravenous isotonic saline:

	1 litre in first 30 mins
then	1 litre in one hour
then	1 litre in two hours

Assess plasma potassium and if below 6 mmol/l then add KCl to subsequent saline infusion.
(d) Intravenous soluble insulin infusion is started immediately at a rate of 5 U/h. When blood glucose falls below 14 mmol/l then change to 4-hourly SC injections of insulin according to urine glucose.
(e) Correct severe acidosis: if blood pH below 7 initially, then give 26 mmol potassium chloride with 100 mmol of sodium bicarbonate intravenously over 30 minutes.

Q5 What are the main types of oral hypoglycaemic agent and how do they act?

A
(a) Sulphonylureas (e.g., glibenclamide) act by stimulating the islets of Langerhans to secrete insulin and by increasing glucose entry into cells.
(b) Biguanides (e.g., metformin) act by inhibiting glucose absorption via the small intestine.

Q6 When are oral hypoglycaemic agents used?

A In adult onset diabetes when diet alone has failed to control the condition.

Q7 When is insulin indicated in diabetes mellitus?

A
(a) When a patient presents with ketosis, polyuria or weight loss – typically in a person under 30 years.
(b) When diet plus oral hypoglycaemic drugs have failed to control the condition.
(c) During critical episodes – especially hyperglycaemic acidosis, operations, infection, ischaemia, trauma, pregnancy and labour.

Q8 What are the absolute contra-indications to the combined oral contraceptive?

A
(a) Thromboembolic disease, phlebitis, coronary artery disease, atrial fibrillation.
(b) Active liver disease.
(c) Known or suspected breast cancer or other oestrogen-dependent tumour.
(d) Undiagnosed cause of vaginal bleeding.
(e) Suspected pregnancy.

Q9 What are the main complications of this method of contraception?

A
(a) Due to oestrogen: thromboembolic disease, migraine, increased capillary fragility, cloasma, increased vaginal mucous discharge, uterine enlargement.
(b) Due to progestogen: depression, fatigue, increased appetite, acne, moniliasis, jaundice.
(c) Due to both agents: hypertension, fluid retention, gallstones, increased mass of breast tissue.

Q10 What is the choice of treatments of thyrotoxicosis?

A
(a) Medical: carbimazole, propylthiouracil, perchlorate.
(b) Surgery.
(c) Radioactive iodine.

Q11 What are the indications for using carbimazole in thyrotoxicosis?

A
(a) Mild to moderate disease – particularly in children, young adults and in the old.
(b) Preparation for surgery.
(c) Thyroid gland not greatly enlarged and not nodular.

Q12 Describe the drug treatment of a thyrotoxic patient prior to partial thyroidectomy.

A
(a) Antithyroid drug: carbimazole.
(b) Propranolol – particularly to reduce tremor and palpitations.
(c) For the 7–10 days before the operation give iodine (as Lugol's iodine) to inhibit release of thyroid hormones.

Both carbimazole and iodine may reduce the vascularity of the gland, and all three drugs reduce the incidence of thyroid crisis.

Q13 Summarise the main dangers of using large doses of glucocorticoids.

A
(a) Cushing's syndrome, wasting of limb muscles.
(b) Associated mineralocorticoid effects: oedema, hypertension, hypokalaemia.
(c) Diabetes mellitus.
(d) Osteoporosis.
(e) Suppression of growth in children with premature fusion of the epiphyses.
(f) Long-term adrenal cortical suppression.
(g) Dyspepsia, aggravation of peptic ulcer.
(h) Depression, mania and other psychoses.
(i) Increased susceptibility to infection.

Q14 Your patient, a girl aged 20 years, suffers from diabetes and requires insulin. She has developed appendicitis and an appendicectomy is planned. How is her diabetes cared for during this crisis?

A
(a) The insulin should be changed to soluble insulin (or analogue) and given 3 times daily if the operation is not to be carried out immediately.
(b) On the day of operation, the blood glucose is measured every 2 hours and the urine is tested for glucose and ketones. Before the operation a 5% glucose intravenous infusion is set up and soluble insulin is given intravenously at a rate of 3 U per hour. The rates of administration of glucose and insulin are

adjusted to prevent ketosis and maintain the blood glucose in the physiological range.

(c) After the operation, when the patient can take food by mouth, the intravenous infusions are stopped and thrice daily injections of soluble insulin are recommenced.

(d) If an infection develops, insulin requirements will increase, even if anorexia and vomiting develop.

Q15 What precautions are required for patients on long-term high dose steroid treatment if they are to undergo surgical operations?

A (a) For major surgery, the patient is given hydrocortisone sodium succinate 100 mg intramuscularly every 6 hours, starting with the premedication and continued until the patient is taking food orally. Hydrocortisone is then given orally 100 mg 6-hourly and then reduced over 7 days. *Pari passu* the patient's usual drug regime is re-introduced.

(b) For minor surgery 100 mg of hydrocortisone sodium succinate is given 6-hourly, intramuscularly for 24 hours.

Q16 How would you manage coma in a lady of 68 who is known to suffer from myxoedema?

A (a) The mortality rate of this condition is high, and the precipitating factors may be complex. The patient is therefore admitted to hospital. The depression in consciousness may be due to lack of thyroid hormones, impaired cerebral circulation, heart failure, hypotension, or lung disease (including severe infection or alveolar hypoventilation).

(b) Tri-iodothyronine is given intravenously (starting with a bolus of 100 μg followed by 20 μg 8-hourly) until the patient starts to recover – usually within 2–3 days.

(c) If the hypothyroidism could be due to pituitary or hypothalamic diseases, hydrocortisone sodium succinate 100 mg intravenously is given 8-hourly.

(d) From the time the patient is first seen, slow rewarming is carried out using metal foil or blankets.

(e) Intravenous fluids are given cautiously, whilst monitoring the central venous pressure. But if heart failure is present, diuretics may be required.
(f) If hypoxia, hypercapnia and respiratory acidosis persist, assisted ventilation may be needed.
(g) If there is a chest infection, then antibiotics are given.

Q17 Outline the treatment of hypercalcaemia.

A (a) The primary cause is looked for.
(b) Intravenous isotonic saline is given to correct dehydration which is often present. Frusemide can be administered concurrently to increase calcium loss.
(c) Hydrocortisone will lower a raised plasma calcium due to malignant disease, sarcoid and vitamin D intoxication.
(d) Calcitonin and mithramycin are both effective in patients with malignant disease involving bones.
(e) Phosphate given orally provides a long-term treatment by binding to dietary calcium in the intestine.
(f) Intravenous chelating agents (such as trisodium edetate) are rarely used. Oral resins, e.g., calcium resonium, are sometimes helpful.

RESPIRATORY SYSTEM

Q1 What are the drugs commonly used in the day-to-day treatment of bronchial asthma?

A (a) Bronchodilators – β agonists, anticholinergics and theophylline. In practice the most useful of these are the selective β_2 agonists inhaled from a metered aerosol. Such drugs include salbutamol, terbutaline and rimiterol.

(b) All patients should have a trial of prophylactic sodium cromoglycate. One cannot predict who will respond well – but this is most likely in children and with asthma which is triggered by allergens, exercise, exposure to cold and to sulphur dioxide. Emotion and infection-triggered asthma is less likely to respond.

(c) Steroids are only used when the above two types of drug do not adequately control the condition. The first strategy with steroids is administration of an aerosol (such as beclomethasone, betamethasone or budesonide) and if this fails then oral prednisolone is given.

Q2 What are the danger signs in an asthmatic which would make you seek specialist advice and/or send him to hospital?

A (a) Sudden failure to respond to the patient's usual bronchodilator aerosol.

(b) Tachycardia and pulsus paradoxicus.

(c) A progressive fall in PEFR.

(d) Inability of the patient to speak a short sentence in one breath.

Q3 Outline the main points in the management of severe refractory asthma (i.e., status asthmaticus).

A (a) Arrange for hospital admission. While waiting for the ambulance to arrive, give 200 mg of hydrocortisone intravenously and if the patient has not been taking a theophylline preparation, give 250 mg of aminophylline intravenously over 5 minutes.

(b) In hospital, set up an intravenous infusion of 5% glucose. Take blood for pH, p_aO_2 and p_aCO_2.

(c) Initial hospital drug therapy may be salbutamol via a facemask and ward nebuliser with oxygen. If the patient has a very low tidal volume, intravenous salbutamol can be given. At this stage intravenous hydrocortisone is also started (e.g., as an infusion of 3 mg/kg/6 h) but it may be up to 4 hours before improvement begins.

(d) Failure to improve is an indication for intubation and positive pressure ventilation.

(e) Antibacterial chemotherapy is not routinely given – but is used if a bacterial infection is suspected.

(f) After 48 hours of intravenous hydrocortisone the steroid is replaced by 80 mg prednisolone orally daily. This is progressively reduced over 10 days.

(g) Sedatives and opioids are absolutely contra-indicated.

Q4 Outline the main therapeutic measures in a patient with acute on chronic bronchitis with emphysema who has secondary heart disease (i.e., cor pulmonale).

A The aim of treatment is to improve alveolar ventilation.

(a) The patient is not receiving enough oxygen and so oxygen is supplied. However patients with CO_2 retention may rely on anoxia as a stimulus to the respiratory centre and giving high concentration oxygen causes respiratory depression with further retention of CO_2. Thus a fixed lower concentration of oxygen (e.g., 24%) is administered via a Venturi-mask. If even this depresses respiration then intermittent positive pressure ventilation is required via a cuffed endotracheal tube.

(b) Bronchospasm is treated with salbutamol inhalation or

injections – sometimes with glucocorticoids as well.

(c) Physiotherapy is important to encourage coughing and increase ventilatory effort. Respiratory stimulants are sometimes given as well but their usefulness is disputed.

(d) Bronchial infection is treated. Amoxycillin or co-trimoxazole are usually appropriate.

(e) Diuretics will improve alveolar ventilation if pulmonary oedema is present.

(f) Digoxin is indicated if there is rapid atrial fibrillation.

(g) Sedatives and opioids are contra-indicated.

ALIMENTARY SYSTEM

Q1 How may drugs assist in the management of peptic ulceration?

A
(a) Antacids (such as aluminium hydroxide) act by neutralising acid and reducing the harmful effect of reflux of bile. These provide symptomatic relief and high dose therapy may accelerate healing.
(b) Histamine H_2 antagonists (cimetidine and ranitidine) accelerate healing by preventing gastrin- and vagal-dependent acid secretion, because histamine acts as the chemical messenger between the histaminocyte and the acid secreting gastric cell.
(c) The resistance of the mucosa may be enhanced by mucus (promoted by carbenoxolone) and by a protective covering (of tripotassium dicitratobismuthate or sucralfate). These agents promote healing.
(d) Anticholinergics such as poldine usually have little beneficial effect but a selective M1 anticholinergic, pirenzepine, accelerates ulcer healing.

Q2 What is purgative abuse?

A Patients who frequently use purgatives may develop abnormalities of intestinal function which include: an atonic colon and increasing dependence on purgatives; water, sodium and potassium loss – sometimes leading to secondary hyperaldosteronism; steatorrhoea and protein losing enteropathy; excessive calcium loss and osteomalacia; dangerous aggravation of other intestinal disease, e.g., an inflamed appendix may rupture.

Q3 What drugs are helpful in ulcerative colitis?

A The treatment can be considered in the two phases of the condition:

(a) In the acute phase prednisolone is the most effective drug. In mild attacks local treatment (e.g., Predsol enemas) may be helpful, but in more severe episodes oral prednisolone is required. In severe refractory illness immunosuppressive drugs (e.g., azathioprine) may be added to the steroid.

(b) In the chronic or inactive stages of the disease sulphasalzine reduces the incidence of relapse. In the chronic phase steroids (local or systemic) may also be needed. Chronic blood loss may cause an anaemia which responds to oral iron. Bran in the diet may control bowel function. Some physicians use codeine to control the diarrhoea. Oral sodium cromoglycate (Nalcrom) has a marginally beneficial effect.

Q4 What types of drug are effective antinausea and antiemetic agents? What are their main clinical uses?

A (a) The neuroleptics block dopamine receptors in the chemoreceptor trigger zone (CTZ) and thus such drugs as prochlorperazine, chlorpromazine and haloperidol are effective in drug-induced vomitting due to CTZ stimulation (e.g., by cytotoxic drugs, opioids, levodopa, bromocriptine), metabolic-induced vomiting (e.g., uraemia) and in terminal illness.

Prochlorperazine may be effective in labyrinthitis.

(b) Metoclopramide and domperidone act on the CTZ and also increase peristalsis in the oesophagus, stomach and small intestine. They are effective in toxin-induced vomiting, drug-induced vomiting (particularly the severe reactions produced by anticancer chemotherapy), postoperative vomiting, migraine and in gastritis.

(c) Anticholinergics, particularly hyoscine, are the most useful agents in travel sickness.

(d) Antihistamines (H_1) such as promethazine, diphenhydramine and cyclizine may also be effective in travel sickness and migraine. So far promethazine has not been associated with fetal abnormalities and thus is used in the sickness of pregnancy. Cyclizine is also used to reduce the nausea caused by opioids.

(e) In the severe nausea due to anticancer treatment, in addition to the previously mentioned drugs, cannabinoids (e.g., nabilone) and prednisolone may be effective.

CHEMOTHERAPY AND RELATED MATTERS

Q1 Which antibiotics are used in the prevention and treatment of subacute bacterial endocarditis?

A (a) For prophylaxis: one hour before dental treatment, patients with damaged heart valves or congenital cardiovascular malformations are given 3 g amoxycillin orally. If the patient is allergic to penicillin, 1.5 g erythromycin is given one hour before treatment and 500 mg is given four times a day for 2 days.

Before a genito-urinary procedure (when *S. faecalis* may be involved), intramuscular ampicillin plus gentamicin are given intramuscularly just before the operation and 12 hours after.

(b) For the treatment of subacute bacterial endocarditis large doses of benzylpenicillin (e.g. 8–20 mega units daily) are given intravenously or intramuscularly if *S. viridans* has been isolated. Blood levels of penicillin are increased by giving probenecid orally.

If *S. faecalis* has been isolated benzylpenicillin with gentamicin are administered intramuscularly. The dose and frequency are modified according to sensitivity results.

Antibiotic treatment of SABE is maintained for at least 6 weeks and until temperature and ESR are normal and embolic phenomena have stopped.

Q2 What are the difficulties in treating hospital staff who are suffering from a *Staphylococcus pyogenes* infection?

A Staphylococcal infections which are acquired in hospital are usually due to organisms which secrete β-lactamase and are therefore resistant to benzylpenicillin and similar penicillins.

These organisms usually respond to β-lactamase-resistant penicillins such as flucloxacillin. The second generation cephalosporins (e.g., cefuroxime) are also relatively resistant to β-lactamase.

Fusidic acid is reserved for such resistant staphylococci. Erythromycin is also usually effective. For patients who are allergic to penicillin, fusidic acid and erythromycin may be used. Such individuals are more likely to exhibit an allergy to cephalosporins as well.

Q3 What are the main uses and hazards of metronidazole?

A Metronidazole is effective against a wide range of anaerobic organisms. These include:

(a) Protozoa – Trichomonas vaginalis infections in men and women
Amoebiasis
Giardiasis

(b) Bacteria – Acute ulcerative gingivitis (Vincent's infection)
Clostridial infections
Non-specific vaginitis (*Haemophilus vaginalis*)

The main hazard is an antabuse-type reaction with alcohol. The drug also causes nausea and metallic taste (it enters the saliva). Fits and headache are uncommon, and metronidazole should not be given if there is active brain disease.

Q4 Which antibacterials can be used for a urinary infection in a pregnant lady?

A The commonest causative organism is *E. coli* although other organisms can cause such an infection. Antifolates (trimethoprim, sulphonamides), nitrofurantoin and tetracyclines cannot be used in pregnancy.

Amoxycillin and ampicillin can be used during pregnancy and are effective against coliforms. Alternative drugs are aminoglycosides and cephalosporins for serious infections if amoxycillin is not suitable, but aminoglycosides are best avoided during pregnancy.

Q5 Outline the treatment of pulmonary tuberculosis.

A Initial investigations and treatment are best carried out by specialists. The patient remains in hospital until the sputum becomes negative for the tubercle bacillus. Sanatorium treatment is no longer carried out.

During the initial two month phase of treatment, four drugs are given daily. These are rifampicin, isoniazid and pyrazinamide plus either ethambutol or streptomycin. The subsequent phase of treatment (usually as an out-patient) consists of daily isoniazid with rifampicin for 4 months. Alternative regimes may be used in which the drugs are given two or three times weekly.

After the initial two month phase, the drug sensitivities of the tubercle bacilli are known, and the drug treatment may have to be modified at that stage.

Q6 What are the biological principles used in designing anticancer chemotherapy?

A (a) A given dose of anticancer drug destroys a constant percentage of malignant cells in unit time. The number of cells surviving after therapy will therefore depend on the size of the tumour mass before treatment. Thus an important principle is to start treatment as soon as possible. Even a few surviving cells can lead to recurrence, so treatment has to be prolonged until the tumour is eradicated.

(b) The other factor which indicates the need for early treatment is that the fraction of dividing cells decreases as the tumour mass increases. As most anticancer drugs act on dividing cells, the tumour will be most susceptible when it is small.

(c) Cytotoxic drugs given repeatedly in short high dose bursts kill more malignant cells than in low doses given continuously. Also the patient's bone marrow recovers more completely in the pauses between treatments and there is also less immunosuppression.

(d) As every tumour cell has to be destroyed it is helpful

if tumour markers (e.g., chorionic gonadotrophin secretion with choriocarcinoma) or sanctuary sites (e.g., testis in lymphoblastic leukaemia) are known so that it is possible to know when to stop treatment.

(e) Combination therapy provides greater therapeutic efficacy than single drugs alone – because the toxic effects are not identical and are therefore not additive in combination. Also, because of differing mechanisms, their action on the neoplasm may be increased and (theoretically at least) the emergence of resistant cells inhibited.

Q7 Summarise the main problems of the immunosuppressed patient.

A (a) Increased susceptibility to infections:
viral: herpes, cytomegalovirus, warts, increased frequency of hepatitis B carriers.
fungal: candida, aspergillus, dermatophytes.
protozoal: pneumocystitis, entamoeba.
bacterial: tubercle, coliforms, pneumococcus.

(b) Increased chance of bacteraemia from certain procedures such as dental treatment, insertion of IUD.

(c) Danger from living vaccines: BCG, yellow fever.

(d) Special problems of individual drugs – thus steroids may cause diabetes, avascular necrosis of bone, osteoporosis, silent perforation of the intestine. Cytotoxics can damage the bone marrow.

(e) Late onset of new tumours, such as lymphomas and skin tumours.

Q8 How would you manage a young man with the signs and symptoms of meningitis, after a lumbar puncture has produced a cloudy CSF under raised pressure? Microscopy shows a large number of polymorphs but no organisms are seen on a direct film.

A (a) The CSF is sent for culture and chemical analysis, but treatment must be started immediately as it is assumed that the patient has meningitis.

(b) Intravenous benzylpenicillin is given in large doses intravenously (e.g., 4 mega U, 6-hourly) and is effective against meningococcus and pneumococcus. At the same time chloramphenicol is given intramuscularly or intravenously in large doses (e.g., 12.5 mg/kg 6-hourly) and is effective against *Haemophilus influenzae*. Penicillin does not readily pass the blood brain barrier, but passage is increased in meningitis. Chloramphenicol does readily enter the CSF and brain.

SOME ASSORTED IMPORTANT TOPICS

Q1 How do you write a prescription for a Controlled Drug for a patient who is not an addict?

A The doctor's name and address must be clearly visible on the prescription.

The rest of the prescription must be in the practitioner's own handwriting in ink and include the date and his signature. The other information must include:

The patient's name and address
The name, form and strength of the drug
The total quantity prescribed (in figures and in words)
The dose

Repeat prescriptions are not allowed.

Q2 Describe the drug treatment of acute anaphylaxis.

A
(a) Intramuscular adrenaline, 0.5 ml of a 1:1000 solution, given early may save life. Oxygen is given.
(b) Intravenous hydrocortisone, 200 mg, is also given as soon as possible. This drug may take 1–3 hours before it starts to exert a beneficial effect on the condition. During this time the adrenaline injection may have to be repeated.
(c) Some physicians would also give an antihistamine such as chlorpheniramine or terfenadine.
(d) If bronchospasm recurs or is not abolished with adrenaline, then intravenous aminophyline 250 mg is given over 5 minutes or salbutamol is given by intravenous injection or by nebuliser and face mask.

Q3 What types of drug may alleviate chronic simple glaucoma?

A
(a) Intraocular pressure is lowered by miotics such as pilocarpine or anticholinesterases (e.g.,

physostigmine), because of opening of the drainage channels in the trabecular network due to contraction of the ciliary muscle. This increases drainage of the aqueous and hence lowers the pressure.

(b) Adrenaline lowers pressure by reducing production of aqueous. Dipivefrin is a prodrug of adrenaline and hence has similar but more prolonged effects. Guanethidine enhances the action of adrenaline.

(c) The β-blocker timolol is very effective in chronic simple glaucoma because it reduces the secretion of aqueous. This drug is contra-indicated in asthmatic patients.

All of the above drugs are given as eye drops.

(d) Acetazolamide is a carbonic anhydrase inhibitor given orally, which also reduces the secretion of aqueous and thus lowers intraocular pressure.

Q4 Summarise the management of psoriasis.

A (a) The patient and his relatives are reassured that the condition is not infectious. All normal activities should be encouraged – including exposure to the sun and swimming.

(b) A common scheme of treatment involves daily tar baths followed by the application of 0.1% dithranol in Lassar's paste to the lesions.

(c) In guttate psoriasis following an acute illness, 3% crude coal tar in a zinc paste or emulsifying ointment can be used all over the skin.

(d) For severe psoriasis specialists may use local fluorinated steroids under polythene occlusion or oral etretinate.

Q5 How are drugs used in the treatment of acne?

A (a) Local treatment involves local cleansing with a detergent followed by a keratolytic such as tretinoin gel, lotion or cream.

(b) Systemic treatment, if required, is long-term, low dose tetracycline or erythromycin. In females cyproterone with ethinyloestradiol (Diane) produces improvement due to its anti-androgenic action.

(c) In severe cystic acne, oral isotretinoin, a vitamin-A derivative, is very effective.

Q6 Indicate the management of co-proxamol (Distalgesic) overdose.

A (a) The initial features are those of acute opioid overdosage due to the dextro-propoxyphene component. Naloxone is an effective antidote and rapidly reverses respiratory depression.

(b) Evidence of paracetamol toxicity may develop days later. As little as 10 g of paracetamol has resulted in severe hepatic (and sometimes renal) necrosis. Antidotes such as acetylcysteine and methionine protect the liver if given within 10–12 hours of ingestion.

Q7 What are the dangers of topical steroids?

A (a) On the skin, local effects include:

(i) skin atrophy – virtually always from potent steroids given for at least 3 weeks.

(ii) infections are made worse and their clinical presentations altered. These include herpes simplex, bacterial infection of eczema, folliculitis, superficial fungal infections and scabies.

(iii) on the face, perioral papular dermatitis and telangiectasia.

(iv) psoriatic lesions may become worse on withdrawal of strong steroids and local or generalised pustular psoriasis may develop.

Enough steroid can be absorbed from the skin to produce systemic effects including growth arrest, adrenal suppression and aggravation of diabetes.

(b) Local steroids inhaled predispose to candida infections of the mouth and pharynx and to hoarseness due to atrophy of the laryngeal muscles.

Q8 What is analgesic nephropathy and how is it managed?

A This is chronic renal damage including renal papillary necrosis, which follows repeated administration of analgesic mixtures. Phenacetin has been implicated, but aspirin and paracetamol and similar mixtures can cause the condition. Perhaps as little as two tablets, three times a day for 3 years may be sufficient in some subjects.

In some surveys, about one fifth of all cases of chronic renal failure are due to this.

Management includes:
prevention (by general publicity of the dangers of analgesic mixtures and advising doctors not to prescribe them);
stopping such drugs if damage has appeared (some improvement in renal function is possible);
treatment of irreversible damage (dialysis or transplant);
treatment of complications (premature ageing and atherosclerosis, renal tract carcinoma, ureteric obstruction).

Q9 Describe the management of nappy rash.

A It is first important to distinguish nappy rash (napkin dermatitis) from atopic eczema, seborrhoeic dermatitis, localised psoriasis and from uncommon serious diseases such as zinc deficiency and histiocytosis X.

The most important preventive and therapeutic measure is a high frequency of nappy changes. Napkin-free times are helpful additional measures. The nappies should be well rinsed and aired after washing. The baby's nappy area is washed with water and *ung. emulsificans*, rinsed, dried and then soft paraffin applied.

Secondary candida infection is treated with mystatin or clotrimazole cream. Mild local steroids are also often used.

Q10 How do you treat a man suffering from a urethral discharge due to a chlamydial infection?

A Assuming that the organism has been positively identified in the laboratory, treatment is started with oxytetracycline 500 mg QDS. Experts differ over how long the treatment should last – some say 3 weeks, but the majority recommend 7 days.

Alternative drugs are doxycycline or minocycline – both given 100 mg BD for 7 days.

The man's sex partner(s) should be treated in the same way, unless a female is pregnant or lactating and breastfeeding, in which case erythromycin 250 mg QDS is given for 14 days.

Q11 How is pediculosis pubis treated?

A Malathion liquid (0.5%) or gamma benzene hexachloride (Lindane application, 0.1%) is applied to the pubic and other hairy areas apart from the scalp, left for one day and then washed off. If Lindane is used, it is repeated after 7 days. The sex partner is treated in the same way.

Q12 How do you treat scabies?

A Gamma benzene hexachloride 1% lotion or cream is applied over the whole body, missing out the head. It is washed off after 24 hours and then repeated after a further 48 hours. The sex partner is treated at the same time. Carbaryl is an alternative treatment.

Q13 How is tricyclic antidepressant overdose managed?

A Gastric lavage is carried out – the anticholinergic properties of these drugs can cause them to remain in the stomach for many hours. Activated charcoal is left in the stomach after it has been emptied.

Depressed respiration may require assisted ventilation. Hypotension and hypothermia may also need treating with plasma expanders and space blankets.

If there are fits, intravenous diazepam is given. Sympathomimetic effects on the heart are treated with β blockers or physostigmine.

Q14 How is aspirin overdose managed?

A Gastric lavage is carried out – but if the patient is conscious, it may be possible to induce vomiting. Aspirin may remain in the stomach for many hours. The patient may be dehydrated, hypokalaemic and acidotic. These conditions can be corrected with intravenous isotonic saline, potassium chloride and sodium bicarbonate. Above a certain plasma level (750 mg/1) forced alkaline diuresis is recommended. Very high plasma levels (above

1000 mg/1) may require haemodialysis or charcoal haemoperfusion.

Sedatives are contra-indicated as these can aggravate acidosis.

Q15 How would you treat a patient with hayfever?

A Mild disease may be managed by avoiding the allergen or by oral antihistamines. Astemizole and terfenadine are much less sedating than the older antihistamines.

Local treatment includes sodium cromoglycate and/or corticosteroids. These should be started 2 or 3 weeks before the start of the hayfever season, because severe mucosal oedema may prevent access of the drugs. Local decongestants (such as ephedrine nose drops) can be used for a short period to facilitate penetration of sodium cromoglycate drops or spray or steroid aerosol, but should not be used for long periods because such vasoconstrictor agents can cause atrophic rhinitis. They can also cause rebound congestion of the nasal mucosa.

Some physicians use systemic corticosteroids for very severe, incapacitating hayfever. Desensitisation may be effective.